Star Dreaming

Star Dreaming

Aunty Bilawara Lee

Senior Aboriginal Larrakia Elders—Healer and Teacher

To order additional copies of this book, contact:
Shrubs Publishing
+61 28006 8158
info@shrubspublishing.com

Table of Contents

Words of wisdom from our Ancestral Grandmother and
Grandfather to help our Spirit journey on the star-paths
back to our celestial family

ACKNOWLEDGEMENTS

Our Ancestral Spirits and Cosmic Grandparents have given me this information and guided me in the writing of this book.

Ian [BEAR] – thank you for your patience and love.

My love and gratitude to my wonderful family, spirit sisters and brothers who have blessed me with love and support and encouragement to put these words of wisdom down on paper.

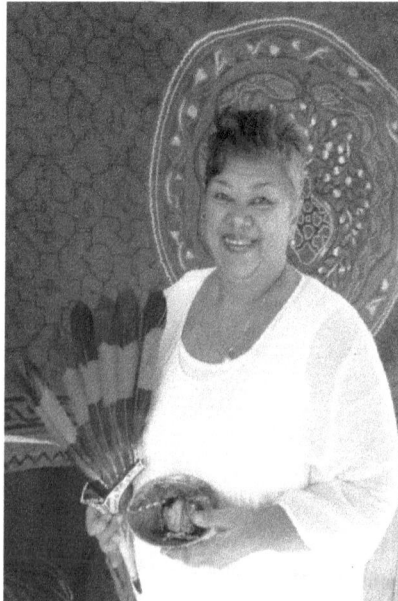

FORWARD

We sit waiting for and wondering when a path will appear for each of us and for us all. Then we hear of Star Dreaming and ask am I supposed to be walking the Star Paths back to our cosmic family? If you are wondering and uncertain then it is time you should hear the words of Bilawara and join us on the journey back to our Cosmic Family.

I am blessed to be apart of such a wonderful story, one that I share with Bilawara and one that our spiritual bond has led me to contribute to this magnificent story channelled by spirit to my spiritual sister and life long friend. When she asked me to write this forward I wondered if I should do it in the traditional manner, but then I was told by spirit to just do it and let it flow, which is what you should do too as you read this book.

Bilawara invited me to contribute to the men's side of this magnificent journey which I do with much reverence. Once you look into this insightful book you will see that it is not a manual for spirituality but more of a guide book for your journey in life and beyond. This book will open your eyes, your mind and your heart to what has been missing in your life. It will help you to connect truly with family and friends and with your community. You will discover that your story does include connection with spirit and that your journey even in this hectic modern world has purpose and even you can live in harmony with each other and the greater world.

Bilawara has given us all a wonderful story, step onto the path and make your own story of your journey into the light.

May the spirits guide you, protect you and support you through this journey.

Anthorr Nomchong

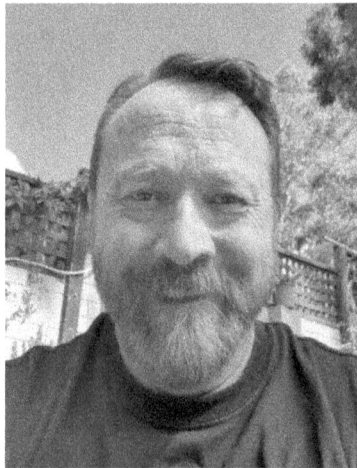

Shaman and Mystic

CHAPTER 1

INTRODUCTION

My name is Auntie Bilawara; it means the red-tailed black cockatoo which is an Ancestral Spirit Being that brings about change, it is my Totem and my Heart Dreaming. I am a Senior Elder of the Larrakia Nation of Darwin Northern Territory, Australia. I am the eldest of 11 children, with seven brothers and three sisters. I have three children and nine grandchildren. I have over 72 years' experience working, living and being a part of a vibrant Aboriginal family and community. I am acknowledged and respected as a Gurdimin-ba Bali – a Spirit Doctor, a healer and teacher of the ancient wisdoms of Aboriginal spirituality and healing.

HISTORY

In 2006 I was blessed with a journey to the United States to join a wonderful group of women at the first International Gathering of Indigenous Grandmothers, acknowledges

Wisdom Keepers of the World. During that visit I was invited to stay with beautiful Jill and her husband Bob in the mountains of Ojai.

In the middle of the night, with a full moon I sat up in bed and began to write. I did not have any lights on and didn't wear my reading glasses. I wrote for quite some time then felt as if I had done what had to be done and went back to sleep.

In the morning I wasn't quite sure that what had happened had really happened until I picked up the exercise book and read my words. I had written most the information for this book. **The Birthing of the White Light Nation:** *Walking the White Light Path*. Since then I have attended three more gatherings and at the last one held in Hawaii the words of wisdoms from our Cosmic Grandparents was sent to me and resulted in **Star Dreaming.**

Since then I have been on a journey of discovery both about myself as the final information for this journey comes through. I have been told that as I am a Grandmother from the oldest, continuing culture on Earth, that it is my role to birth the newest. So come walk with me along the star paths.

CHAPTER 2

THE JOURNEY

Over many years of travelling speaking and teaching many people about Aboriginal spirituality and healing I have had the opportunity to observe others seeking enlightenment and to witness many disturbing events.

I saw, met and spent time with many beautiful people from not only Celtic and European traditions but from many different mixed racial heritage, who for whatever reason have been disconnected from their own cultural rituals and ceremonies and who are actively seeking teachers of ancient wisdoms – Indigenous people who could help them on their path of spiritual enlightenment. One of the most common statements made to me is that they "didn't have any spiritual history" and that they had lost all their connection to cultural ritual and ceremonies and it was obviously a painful state to be in.

Unfortunately, I see many people become victims of abuse from members of the red, black and yellow nations and by people portraying themselves as teacher, shamans, medicine men and false prophets. There is a growing energy of arrogance that the yellow, black or red nations are somehow better because of their history of suffering and ongoing connection to "Spirit" and people of these nations are able to continue to perform their rituals and ceremonies. Many people have come to believe that they don't have a connection to spirit and don't have any of their own rituals, ceremonies and beliefs.

This has led to the dimming and almost extinction of the white light energy that is so important for the overall spiritual wellbeing of humanity.

I pass on the information given to me by the Ancestors and I hope it helps you with your journey to becoming a higher being.

When we all stand in a circle, the red, black and yellow nations stand confident and strong but the white light nation does not share that state of being so I call on my brothers and sisters from the red, black and yellow nations to support and nurture the white light nation on its journey.

ALL OF MANKIND IS EVOLVING INTO THE ONE RAINBOW NATION – ONLY THEN CAN WE CAN BECOME THE CRYSTAL NATION AND THEN THE STAR NATIION

LOVE KNOWS NO BOUNDARIES

LOVE YOURSELF AND THE PLANET WILL BE
HEALED

LISTEN TO THE WISDOM OF THE ANCESTORS
AND BEWARE OF FALSE PREACHERS AND
PROPHETS

The white Light Nation must stand in its own 'power' / energy / vibration as we cannot have a rainbow without white light. The red, black and yellow nations are practicing spiritual rituals and ceremonies but many others have not yet united. If there is no white light nation we will all fail. This a critical time and the white light people must catch up or they will be left behind.

Being a member of the White Light Nation and on the white light path is not restricted to the colour of a person's skin – it is the essence of your heart. Anyone can choose this path and just because you are white skinned doesn't mean you must follow this path if you are already happy following one of the spiritual paths of another nation.

BACKGROUND

For the ancients, spirituality was a shared responsibility, with both sexes acknowledged for their individual strengths and weaknesses on an equal basis. Spirituality was not something to be labelled. It was a way of life. It was what one did to live a healthy, abundant life. It was realised that for the Earth Mother and the Creator Spirit to continue to supply the people with what was required for them to survive, they had to honour the source, live in harmony with Nature and treat each other with love and respect. They also realised that what is given had to be acknowledged and offered back to the Earth in a sacred way.

Men are equally as aware as women, but since time was new, women have taken to the intuitive arts quicker and on a much easier, more natural level, and men have been allowed to forget. We hear about the phases of the Moon and the three phases of women as maiden, mother and crone, but, what of the youth, father and sage? What of the god aspect: the male consort to the goddess? Many men have forgotten what it means to be a real male, as apposed to a 'real man', while many women are striving to remember what it means to be a woman.

In ancient times, it was the women who dreamed the future and determined the path of the people. It was the women who visioned where the best hunting and gathering places were to be found and the safest ground to set up camp. It was the women who governed the people, and they did so by trusting their intuition and their connection to Spirit.

It was the men, though, who took these dreams and visions to the Creator Spirit and asked for signs as to how they should be brought to fruition. The men trusted Spirit because they trusted their women. They knew that neither would let them down, because they trusted their own Spirit and knew their Purpose and who they were in the bigger scheme of things. The men honored the menstrual blood as the driving force of life, and saw the bleeding of the women as a sacred time of immense power. In the days of our ancestors, the men and the women worked hand in hand. Their lives were interwoven on all levels. There was balance. They complemented each other physically, spiritually and emotionally and they supported and compensated one another's weaknesses.

Women were once seen as messengers of the spirit realms, fulfilling the role of the keepers of love magic, prophet, healer, educator and philosopher. Men have always been the active ones: the developers, hunters and collectors, the foot soldiers and defenders. Despite these clearly defined roles, both men and women once gathered in sacred counsel. They may have gathered separately or at individual power times, but when they did, they stood opposite while honoring the other as a balancing force and equal in their own right. The women dreamed and shared their visions with the men, who sat collectively at peace within their role as the ones expected to consciously bring them to fruition. Although the women were the ones who visioned the future, the men were the ones who harnessed the energy and manifested the outcome. Vibrationally, masculine energy is insubstantial in form and cannot be held within the palm of one's hand. Masculine energy is generally witnessed or experienced rather than being physically contained. The warmth of the Sun, the passion created by an intimate encounter, the violence of war; all these occurrences are energetically experienced and are therefore masculine in form. Feminine energy, however, is tangible and real to the touch. The experiences had within the womb, the birthing of children; the ever-changing cycles of nature and the growing and eventual harvesting of the crops are all energetically feminine in their form. They are physical experiences that can be bodily explored and recorded by the senses. The ancients knew this, and celebrated the fact on a daily basis in both ritual and ceremony as well as in their day-to-day lives. It was real, practical and afforded them great power. It was the way life was meant to be lived.

Men and women must walk together; the separation of the genders has caused an imbalance which needs to be rectified. The other nations (red, black and yellow) must start to walk together with the white light nation, and together we must all walk together equally as men and women.

We need to celebrate our existence here on Earth as spiritual beings having a physical experience.

It is time for us to encourage our mothers, sisters and daughters to continue to learn physical skills, advance academically and consider them-selves capable, if not more so, of achieving everything that their brothers can, while maintaining their ability to vision, honor their Moontime and commune directly with Spirit/Mother Earth.

It is time for us to encourage our fathers, brothers and sons to cry, love, dream, trust their intuition and sing from their hearts while still becoming the solid, grounded provider/protector and/or warrior Spirit as Mother Earth intended them to be.

CHAPTER 3

*E*ach of us is a spiritual being, we live in a body and we possess a soul. We are on a spiritual journey and must do the journey without soul influences

BODY SOUL SPIRIT

Body

This is your PHYSICAL being. It is flesh made from a collection of mineral elements and is mostly water. It is born, grows, matures, begins to deteriorate and eventually dies, and then decomposes back into its basic elements and remains a part of the dust of the world. The body is a part of you but is NOT ALL of what defines who YOU are.

When we die the body goes back to Mother Earth

Soul

- Is the combination of mind, intellect, will, emotions, physical feeling and desires – it performs rational and intellectual functions
- The soul is what causes you to cling to the material world and materialism
- The soul is what causes you to display emotions

- The soul is behind the scene watching and influencing, controlling the mind and body – it is what decides when to resist urges, to fight tendencies.
- The soul can gather negativity which will weigh the spirit down – slowing its journey. If the soul is not weighed down by negativity and is light - it will support the spirits journey
- The soul is what we call **consciousness or ego**

The soul dies with the body. The only difference is when you live a life of love and compassion your soul merges with your spirit and you have past life memories.

Spirit

- The Spirit is the energy that fills a person, it is the astral or cosmic body – it is the network of energy channels or "song-lines" – ley-lines or dreaming tracks within the physical body. The Spirit is solid energy – your aura or essence.
- The Spirit is the source of power and control for both your body and soul – it can be either evil or good, darkness or light, unclean or clean – positive or negative.
- The Spirit or "breath of life" is eternal. The spirit has no need for emotions, desires or sinfulness – Our Spirit comes from the creator - from the beginning - and continues on its journey of enlightenment striving to become a being of a higher order

The spirit does not die with the body and continues on its journey to the stars.

YOU MUST LIVE WITH UNCONDITIONAL LOVE AND AN OPEN HEART CHAKRA

With Mother Earth's vibration rising and with the changes that are already taking place, we must live with our hearts open and loving. There is energy from the stars already falling to Earth (I see it as star dust – glittery sparkles in the air). Soon there will be much more. To be able to work with, filter or channel the star dust you must have an open heart. The heart is the major organ in our bodies, the only organ that can work with this cosmic energy – anyone who is unable or unwilling to open their hearts will no longer be able to remain on Mother Earth. Just as our lungs allows us to breath and the other major organs allows us to live. As we are a spiritual being, coming from the beginning with the ancestors and travelling to the stars, an open heart will nurture and support your spiritual journey.

I see "star dust" coming from the cosmic Ancestors as fuel for our spiritual journey. Just as you have the fuel pump opening in your car to received fuel to allow the car to move. Our heart is the body's opening to allow the "star dust" fuel to be taken in so it can fuel our spiritual journey.

CHAPTER 4

CHANGES

Today we are facing a new Era. The ancient Mayan culture speaks of this change, the ending of their old calendar in 2012, and the beginning of a new age. They, along with many other Indigenous cultures, also speak that these times as one of a more feminine nature, based in the heart and unconditional love.

But people in our modern world have a problem. We have begun to become financially and professionally empowered. Yet the most important need, for spiritual empowerment, is often neglected or ignored.

Our world is already in the time of transition and it will be a difficult time until the new era blossoms into an age of peace and understanding. If our world is to survive, spiritually empowered men and women must take their place in helping. It's time for us to step up and step out. The time of hiding is over.

Most "aware" people know that it is necessary to heal our Mother Earth if we are to survive. However, it is equally as imperative to also heal ourselves and each other through unconditional love, compassion and respect. Moreover, women also need to help our men and boys develop their own feminine aspects of gentleness and sensitivity, compassion, nurturing, and kindness. We need to help our male counterparts learn to work from the heart. Men you need to help your women to become stronger and less dependant on others.

It won't be easy but if we don't do all of this, we can't help our planet and humanity risks extinction.

People of earth-based knowledge and wisdoms, take courage. You carry the teaching of our Ancestors and people will look to you for guidance. Be mindful of your walk.

You are the ones we have been waiting for. It's time to step up. And yes, I'm speaking to each of you.

False Prophets

Currently there is a waves of false prophets coming forth, they are connected to the dark ley lines, negative energy and the hold themselves up as medicine people, prophets, shamans etc. and looking to implant their negative energies in those who have forgotten their humility, people who are anchored in their soul journey, not spirit journey and are blind. So these energies take over a person's core without them knowing it. How do we detect these false prophets? They still appear to radiate light and speak "light" but also project false humility and find ways to promote themselves, they demonstrate a need to dominate, to be seen as the "guru" and make a lot of money with their so called words of wisdom.

Solution: send those that are "blind" compassion and unconditional love. They have forgotten their way. We need to be the light sources that are catalysts to bring them back home. So it's a delicate balancing act and the need to be clear and strong spiritual warriors in the process. Here is a ritual that came to me from our Cosmic Grandparents which can help you work with those that are "blind".

Dragonfly Meditation

In most Indigenous cultures around the world the dragonfly represent the bringing in of light, so it was appropriate that I was given this mediation to help those who had lost the ability to "see".

Smudge/balance/ground/protect/filter *(these rituals can be found further in the book)*.

- See yourself sitting quietly in a special place.
- See yourself blanketed with sparkling little starlight dragonflies.
- See them come one by one to kiss you and then fly off across the earth.

- See each little starlight dragonfly go to people who are stumbling around in the dark.
- See a starlight dragonfly bring some light into their lives – it will help them see clearly the false prophets and enable them to get back on the star paths for their spiritual journey.

CHAPTER 5

STAR DREAMING INFORMATION

This information was given to me to pass on to you all. It helps you place yourself in the energy of Star Dreaming.

- Wear white for rituals, particularly the birthing ceremony – you don't have to be in total white, just a shirt/blouse or skirt/trousers, scarf etc.
- Wear garlands of rainbow/multi coloured flowers/crystals, beads, ribbons around head, neck, waist, wrist etc.
- Sacred number 8 – the infinity symbol. The infinity symbol is rainbow coloured and represents Mother Earth's [ME] girdle/belt [song-line] and resonates with Mother Earth's energy vibration.
- Carry staffs [can put anything on it]; white light nation members should make their own in whatever wood they like.

- The energy of the star paths is gentle, the sound of small bells and chimes. It is the energy of moonstones, clear quartz crystal and starlight. The vibration of the White Light Nation is a flowing, gentle movement which includes sparkling starlight and gossamer energy
- Honour the animals, they will walk with us – and often their give-away sacrifice for us to survive is done with unconditional love. The animals are here to teach us unconditional love. Messages from the spirit world can be transmitted through animals – to us and from us. When we become the Rainbow Nation the animals will be part of that. Working with different animal totems can assist for certain situations and everyone should get to know what the different energy is for each animal.
- We and the animals are rainbow bridges.
- Listen to the children – any child born since 1985 have been born with extra DNA and see things more five dimensional than three so can help those of us who are older – they are further along the path to becoming a part of the crystal nation.
- Live simply [do not be materialistic], people on the star paths will not need "things" or possession to be happy and productive. The more you know the less you need.
- Honour the environment - grow your own food, which will resonate with your own 'song' or energy – much more nutritious and better for you

- Must live with your heart chakra open – with unconditional love and compassion
- Cleanliness is important, you must keep your body, mind, spirit, soul and the environment clean and healthy. Washing cleanses the body, prayer cleanses the soul and the 'smudging/smoking' ritual cleanses the spirit. The smudging/smoking ceremony is particularly important.
- Modesty in clothing [no bums, boobs, midriffs, knees or see-through]. The current trend to "hang' everything out for public viewing only stimulates the groin chakra, which detracts from the opening of the heart chakra, therefore encouraging people to live a soul journey not a spirit journey.
- must let go of the energy of:

    o dominance
    o superiority – being too prideful
    o jealousy
    o being judgemental
    o being competitive
    o being ego-centric
    o being over dramatic
    o being greedy
    o hanging on to old hurts, resentment, anger, hate etc

- Be aware of your [WATCH]:

    o **Words**

- o **A**ctions
- o **T**houghts
- o **C**onduct
- o **H**eart

You can physically attack/harm other people though your words, actions, thoughts, conduct and heart. You can also be harmed by others in this way.

- NO
  - o Drugs
  - o Alcohol
  - o Tobacco
  - o Addictions

You must not use any of the above as it disconnects you from our spirit guides and ancestral beings and hinders your spiritual growth, abilities and journey.

- Healer heal thyself, we must get our 'song'/vibration in tune with Mother Earth [ME]. Each vibration has a colour; Mother Earth's [ME] vibration is rainbow and she is evolving to crystal white light.
- Your personal vibration/'song' must be in tune so you can sing in harmony with Mother Earth's [ME] songline
- Mother Earth, Father Sun. Grandmother/Grandfather moon. Grandmother is full moon, Grandfather is dark moon

- Individually we must clean up our environment. Take care of the survival of yourself and our immediate family.

Food growing

- Learn how to grow your own food or establish a network with others so you can barter for food
- Keeping domestic animals such as chickens
- Security – safe natural homes with independent power sources such as solar panels
- Learn about your local native bush foods and bush medicines
- Learn a skill – eg: making candles, working with leather, making soap, cutting hair, healing or massage. This could be used to barter for other goods or services.

- People on the star paths must take care of your brothers and sisters from the Black, Yellow and Red Indigenous nations as they are also part of the Rainbow Nation. They know how to survive – you will need them to survive the coming Mother Earth [ME] changes – they are still deeply connected to Mother Earth and the plant and animal kingdoms.
- Brothers and sisters from the Black, Yellow and Red Indigenous Nations must nurture and support anyone who wants to be on the stars paths.

CHAPTER 6

FUNDAMENTAL RITUALS FOR WELLBEING

To help you on your spiritual journey, I have set out below some fundamental rituals that have been taught to me as a child and have never stopped performing as I know they work. These rituals have kept me on my star path, protected, guided and supported. These I now share with you.

SMOKING CEREMONY

All cultures use smoke as a spirit cleanser.

Water cleanses your body – meditation and prayer cleanse your soul and ritual smoke cleanses your spirit.

Many Indigenous communities use different plants from their particular region for the smoking ritual.

- Different peoples from many different diverse cultures use different plants for their "smoking" ceremonies.

- Currently sage, lavender, cedar, sweet-grass, frankincense or myrrh has a beautiful gentle energy when used for the smoking ceremony.
- Wormwood currently burns with the perfect 'energy' for today's needs – it kicks butt!

Smoking will:

- Cleans the spirit of all negativity, which sticks and becomes heavy and can sometimes be seen as a dark mass on someone's shoulders. Negativity sticks to the soul and slows down the spirits journey.
- Sever all 'tentacles' people (friends, family and colleagues) put on us. These tentacles are used to 'push' and 'pull' us around. Severing these tentacles allows us to be independent, 'walk our talk' and live our lives without influences. We can then take full responsibility for our actions and outcomes.
- Cleanses our environment of negativity and evil/heavy energies.
- Anyone with a hidden agenda will not be able to enter your cleansed space or will be become very uncomfortable even sick if they do.
- Will help protect you from psychic attack.
- Should be the start of all healing sessions or rituals and ceremonies.
- Smoking an object given to you will also dissolve all 'obligations' attached to that gift.

- People smoke a place when someone dies. Smoking heals and purifies people - it enters them and strengthens them when they feel sad or weak.

GROUNDING:

Connects you to Mother Earth and prevents you from being "thrown" off balance by any sudden or traumatic experiences. Allows you to be stable and in control and therefore cannot be influenced by negative energies and influences. Will allow you to be sensitive both physically and spiritually to the ebb and flow of energies in your environment and will allow Mother Earth to nurture, support and protect your spiritual journey.

- Smudge/smoke yourself in the spirit cleaning ceremony
- Sit, preferably outside, place your bare feet on Mother Earth.
- Visualise your energy flowing deep down into Mother Earth and then flowing out just like tree roots, which will anchor you solidly.
- Allow your energy to flow upwards and outwards so that you can 'sense' the energy flows around you. This can also give you warning if there is any danger from another person, raising your awareness of your place in the environment. You can 'pull' in your energy at any time when you feel you need to protect yourself.

BALANCING [this can follow immediately after grounding]

Balancing will assist in keeping your emotions serene and moving along in a gentle wave like motion – your emotions won't become scattered and you will be very aware of everything tangible and intangible in your life.

- Smudge/smoke yourself in the spirit cleaning ceremony
- Close your eyes and sense your inner self/core – like a small solid ball of you that floats around inside you body
- Pull that solid ball of your inner self/core down to just below your navel and anchor there.
- Once balanced you should be able to withstand being pushed by someone or by a traumatic event. You should be able to stand solid and not stumble or fall over when shocked by being pushed or traumatised.

PROTECTION [*this can follow immediately after Balancing*]

Protection is critical for your total wellbeing. To remain strong, healthy and safe you must protect yourself from outside influences, particularly false prophets.

- Smudge/smoke yourself in the spirit cleaning ceremony
- Visualise a bubble completely around yourself made of something reflective, such as water.
- The reflective side of the bubble must be positioned away from your body so that anything "sent" at you (such as a psychic attack or negative energy) will be reflected away from you.

- The bubble can be in any colour.
- Outside the layer of bubble, place a filter so that only positive energy can flow into the bubble. The filter will siphon out any negative energy. Visualise three separate pyramids with the outer pyramid with holes which allow white light energy in – then the middle pyramid with smaller holes which allow the nearly completely filtered white light through then the final, most inner pyramid will only allow pure, clean white light energy through to nurture your spirit. All negativity will have been siphoned off.

FILTERING

Once you have done the other rituals you must then put up filters so that when you channel energy to do spiritual work you must only allow white light/goodness or positive energy to enter. To just open up and start energy work is very dangerous as you can also attract negative, dark energy and if you don't have filters in place then you can become sick or infected with dark light.

- Visualise yourself with a series of filters outside your protective bubble. I personally see three eight sided stars with each progressive inner star with smaller and smaller "holes" in them until only white light can come through. Any darkness is filtered away.

SINGING MOTHER EARTHS'S SONGLINES

Singing the Mother Earth's Songline is silent – not verbal, not aloud, so when you want to harmonise with Mother Earth's vibration – sit in silence and "sing" with your own personal energy. Rest or meditate - by moving silently across the earth you "sing" energy and love to Mother Earth's vibration and this helps make the earth, animals and environment strong and healthy.

Singing Mother Earth's Songlines in Silence will disconnect your soul and engage your spirit and it will:

- Allow the animal kingdom to <u>support</u> your song
- Allow the crystal kingdom to <u>amplify</u> your song
- Allow the plant kingdom to <u>nurture</u> your song
- Allow the Cosmos and ancestral spirits to <u>protect</u> your song

CHAPTER 7

**RITUALS FOR STAR DREAMING FOR
STAR DREAMING MEMBERS**

1. Birthing and Naming ceremony
2. Sprouting ceremony
3. Star flow-time/Becoming a man
4. Marriage/commitment
5. Honouring the Parents and Childbirth
6. Star Fire - Menopause or becoming the Crone or Sage
7. Becoming and Elder
8. Death

**THE BIRTHING CEREMONY – NAMING
CEREMONY**

- Big long white arch, made out of natural products such as wood, branches etc, covered in white things: flowers, feathers, ribbon, bells, chimes, crystals beads. Must be high enough for people to walk through. The arch must be biodegradable – so it can go back to Mother Earth

- The men and women who are being 'birthed' sit and work together to make the arch. They dress in white when being birthed.
- Eight couples representatives from the four different 'tribes' [black, white, red and yellow] will stand at the opening of the arch to usher the new person through the arch – the Grandmother will stand at the other opening to welcome the birthed person into the tribe/onto the white path. Grandmother will wear purple.
- A "Smoking Ceremony" will be done before the people being birthed walked through the tunnel/arch.
- A celebration is then held

THE SPROUTING CEREMONY—FEMALE RITUAL

Women gather together with the young woman, they sing songs and dance and eat together; the older women instruct the younger woman about life and love magic. It is a gentle ritual, a time of bonding and initiation for the young woman into the women's circle.

STAR FLOW TIME

Starflow: the young woman is taken to a special place and looked after by the women especially Grandmother/s. A smoking ceremony is held for everyone and a time of celebration begins. The young woman is given instructions about her body and about the sacred journey of star flow time. It is the time for dreaming and prophecy. A small intimate party is held and the young woman receives gift from the other women.

The young woman is given instructions on the three phases of women as maiden, mother and crone. She learns about the responsibility of dreaming the future and determining the path of the people, about trusting her intuition and their connection to Spirit/Mother Earth. Moontime is a sacred time of immense power.

The Grandmother/s will instruct the young woman on how to encourage and support their men; how to drop expectations and realise that their men are largely innocent (not ignorant) to the ways of Spirit/Mother Earth and that they need time, love and patience if they are to catch up.

BECOMING A MAN—MENS RITUAL

Becoming a Man:_ At an agree time a young man is taken to a special place by the men and Grandmother/s. A smoking ceremony is held for everyone and a time of celebration begins. A small intimate party is held and the young man receives gifts from the other men.

The young man is given instructions on the three stages of a man's life – youth, father and sage. He gets instructions on the god aspect: the male consort to the goddess. What it is to be a real male as apposed to being a "real man". He learns about his role to take the dreams and visions from the women and take them to the Creator Spirit and how to ask for signs as to how they should be bought to fruition. He is encouraged to trust Spirit because he must learn to trust the women. He learns about Starflow time and how he must honour the menstrual blood as the driving force of life. He must see the moon-time of the women as a sacred time of immense power.

The Grandmother will instruct the young man about woman and their physical and spiritual journeys, including Moontime, childbirth and women's intuition. They will give the young man instructions on how to show their love and appreciation to their women and children and therefore how to love themselves.

MARRIAGE/COMMITMENT

A self designed marriage/commitment ceremony can be done in partnership with a Civil Celebrant and Elder/Spiritual Leader.

Have the ritual in a special place (preferably outdoors). The couple to wear white and must write their own vows, which will be spiritual and legal heart of the ceremony.

The Celebrant/Elder/Spiritual Leader can wear purple or rainbow colours.

The ceremony can include song, dance, cultural rituals and the exchange of rings. This is entirely up to the couple, whatever will make the event special to them.

The Smoking Ceremony must be done at the beginning of the wedding ceremony and at the end the Authorised Marriage Celebrant/Elder/Spiritual Leader can do a wedding blessing (and if done by an Indigenous Elder, a blessing from the Ancestors).

A feast can be held with family and friends.

HONOURING THE PARENTS AND CHILDBIRTH

An honouring the parents ceremony is a wonderful alternative to the traditional 'baby shower' that is held for parents approaching birth. Parents should invite those people closest to them, in whose friendship and wisdom they trust. You can invite friends to bring a plate of food and/or a gift if you like, but a special ceremony as part of your day is the central feature of the ritual. It is a time of receiving for the parents to be, a time where you are nurtured and honoured by your community.

The Honoring the parents ceremony acknowledges the commitment and energy involved in being parents. This ceremony can be given to the parents each time they have a child, as with each child comes a new level of commitment and surrender. The key is for the 'parents to be' to allow yourself to receive and 'fill your cup' as deeply as possible. The ceremony is also a powerful way to assist in the parent's preparation for birth. It gives others present in the circle the opportunity to share the experiences. Often it is a time when the 'parents to be' can express any fears or worries in a safe and sacred setting and receive the support they need.

NAMING CEREMONY:

This ceremony is a fulfilling and meaningful experience for all concerned. It is an occasion where a new birth is celebrated and a child is welcomed into the world. Family relationships are deepened and parents become more fully aware of their responsibilities. So, too, do the grandparents and godparents/guardians/mentors.

The naming ceremony is an excellent occasion for the cultural expression of joy, hope and acceptance. Every aspect of the naming ceremony can be personalised to suit your personal situation. The ceremony must reflect you as a parent (one or two), your style, your feelings, aims, dreams and wishes for your child. The introduction, the prose, poetry, verse, music, lyrics and/or choreography must reflect to the best of your ability who you are and what you want for your child.

Most often naming ceremonies are held in or around the home, a meaningful expression of nurturing, love and togetherness. As small children are often present in the form of siblings, cousins or friends of the family, the family home is often the safest, most practical and convenient place to have a ceremony.

Choosing a name for a child is an important part of the birthing process. Having a ceremony to mark this occasion can be a celebration of the new life and a welcome, recognition of parenthood and a time of sharing and strengthening of friendships.

When children are adopted, fostered, or become part of a step family a naming ceremony is a wonderful way of welcoming them into their new or extended family.

PLACENTA CEREMONY

A ceremony is done with the Placenta, by planting it under a plant, flower (you can choose any plant or bush that you like) to return them back to the source. Planting the placenta, with honour and awareness, was returning back to the source the memory of our time in the Universal Star Matrix. The Ancestors teach that our birth is our first ceremony on this planet. In the old days, it was witnessed, celebrated, and was a way to make sacred this connection to our Mother Earth and our origins from the Stars.

Each family and friend would out loud, announce each child to the Universe and the world - dedicating a blessing to help the children as they grow. This is a lovely way to celebrate the baby's introduction to Mother Earth.

STAR FIRE - MENOPAUSE/BECOMING THE CRONE or SAGE

The Crone

Star-fire

When a woman goes through menopause and has hot flushes. She needs to "pull" the heat from her groin to her heart and then channel the energy to Pele (Goddess of Fire) who will send the "fire of love energy" down into Mother Earth's core. The stardust that is being sent to us by our Cosmic Grandparents that carries the love energy is being sent as Mana (from heaven) from our Cosmic Grandmother and Grandfather. It not only fuels our spirits but the spirit of Mother Earth who is so parched.

The combination of stardust/love energy and fire from Pele [star-fire energy] and the Circle of Elders conducting the Seed Dreaming ceremony [planting the seeds of change] humanity will be able to walk the star-paths home.

In early cultures, the female elder was considered a wise woman. She was the healer, the teacher, the imparter of knowledge. She mediated disputes, she had influence over tribal leaders, and she cared for the dying as they took their final breaths. For many women in Wicca and other Pagan religions, reaching the status of Crone is a major milestone. These women are reclaiming the name of Crone in a positive way, and see it as a time to joyfully welcome for one's position as an elder in training within the community.

A Croning ceremony may be performed by an Elder/Spiritual Leader, but can also be performed by other women who have already attained the position of Crone. The ceremony itself is typically performed as part of a women's circle or gathering.

Friends and family come together to build an arch or tunnel for the ceremony, the arch/tunnel should be made of natural material and decorated with white objects such as flowers, ribbons, feathers, stars or crystals. Other young women would escort the initiate to the opening of the arch/tunnel and the Crone to be would walk through to be greeted at the other end by other Crones, and therefore be initiated into the Circle of Crones.

There are no set rules for how a ceremony is conducted, but many women who have achieved the title of Crone find they like to include at least some of the following:

- A ritual bath or cleansing beforehand – dress in white
- Smoking Ceremony
- Music with singing and chanting
- Symbols of initiation -- a staff, a special cloak, a garland or crown
- The passage through the arch/tunnel into Cronehood -- entering through a tunnel and crossing a ceremonial threshold into the Crone circle
- An exchange of gifts or blessings (a Croning basket filled with chocolates and herbal teas is popular)
- A celebratory meal can be held

Some women choose to adopt a new name at their Croning Ceremony -- this is certainly not mandatory, but just as we take new names for other milestones in our lives, if you feel that this is right for you, do so. Your Crone name can be one you keep to yourself, share only among friends, or announce to the world.

The Sage—Men's ritual

As with the Crone, becoming the Sage is the time for a man to decide what legacy he will leave to the world and a time to pass on wisdom and experiences to others, especially the young males (warriors) in his community. This is also the beginning of the time to prepare himself to become an Elder.

A Sage ceremony may be performed by an Elder/Spiritual Leader, but can also be performed by other men who have already attained the position of Sage. The ceremony itself is typically performed as part of a men's circle or gathering.

Friends and family come together to build an arch or tunnel for the ceremony, the arch/tunnel should be made of natural material and decorated with white objects such as flowers, ribbons, feathers, stars or crystals. Other young men (warriors) would escort the initiate to the opening of the arch/tunnel and the Sage-to-be would walk through to be greeted at the other end by other Sages, and therefore be initiated into the Circle of Sages.

There are no set rules for how a ceremony is conducted, but many men who have achieved the title of Sage find they like to include at least some of the following:

- A ritual bath or cleansing beforehand – dress in white
- Smoking Ceremony
- Music with singing and chanting
- Symbols of initiation -- a staff or a special cloak – any gifts of knowledge and wisdom
- The passage through the arch/tunnel into Sagehood -- entering through a tunnel and crossing a ceremonial threshold into the Sage circle -- entering through a curtain or tunnel, crossing a ceremonial threshold
- An exchange of gifts or blessings
- A celebratory meal can be held

BECOMING AND ELDER

Crossing the threshold into becoming an Elder can be a major event in a person's life. It's a celebration of all that you've learned, and all that you will come to know in the future. For many, it's a time to make new commitments and vows. If you've ever had an interest in taking a leadership position in some aspect of your life, now is a great time to do so. This seventh cycle of your life is the one in which you become an Elder, and you've joined a special group. You have a lifetime of achievements behind you, and decades more to look forward to. The word Elder should now be a word of power for you, so celebrate it. You've earned it.

A gathering is held with friends and family to celebrate the graduation to Wise Woman or Wise Man. The "This is Your Life" style event can include:

Song, dance, music and gifts to the person become the wise one. Friends and family can stand and give acknowledgment and respect to the Wise one with stories about their life and accomplishments.

- A ritual bath or cleansing beforehand – dress in white
- Smoking Ceremony
- Singing and music
- Gifts of love and acknowledgements for the person's life journey
- A symbol of the passage into becoming an Elder – being led to the tunnel by other Crones and Sages then entering through a tunnel to be greeted by other Elders at the end
- An exchange of gifts or blessings of love for the Elders life journey
- A feast can be held to celebrate the occasion.

DEATH

The passing of a member of the community is not only a time of sadness but of joy also as the deceased has completed their journey in this life and their spirit is moving on to their next journey. When a spirit crosses over they join the circle of Ancestors and will still be there to be with you, just in a different form. The Spirit or "breath of life" is eternal. The spirit has no need for emotions, desires or sinfulness – Our Spirit comes from the creator - from the beginning - and continues on its journey of enlightenment striving to become a being of a higher order.

- Close friends and family lovingly prepare the body for burial.
- Conduct a Smoking Ceremony for everyone
- Family and friends gather for the funeral where they can speak about the deceased with words of love and acknowledgement of their life.
- Music with singing and chanting
- Funeral ceremony conducted by civil celebrant or priest
- When the coffin has been placed in the ground, friends and family to cover the coffin with flowers and flower petals before the hole is filled in.
- Elder/Spiritual Leader to give a Blessing from the Ancestors.
- A celebratory meal can be held

CHAPTER 8

CLOSING INFORMATION

Ceremonies are a Fundamental Need

Life is a continual spiritual, emotional, mental and physical journey in constant change. Our lives are our Spirit's - Sacred Life Journey. Our Journey is inseparable from Mother Earth with all her life forms and energies. Our thoughts and beliefs are inseparable from Divine Creation. Everything in this dimension is divinely conscious.

Ceremonies are an essential foundation, a universal human need that heals and celebrates the union of our Divine Consciousness with Divine Mother Earth Creation. Ceremonies create a greater ease and grace of life's changes, passages and expansion of our own personal and spiritual growth.

Ceremonies create a strong sacred inner link that assists us to easily surf all the unexpected and unknown waves, great tsunamis and great life mysteries of both our outer and inner landscapes.

With Ceremony, balance and harmony are restored in our lives of our shared sacred breath of life, the sacred breath of the Divine Source Love we all share.

STAR DREAMING POEM

Love

True love is neither physical nor romantic;
True love is an acceptance of all this is, has been, will be and will not be;
The happiest people don't necessarily have the best of everything;
They just make the best of everything they have;
Life is not about how to survive the storm; but how to dance in the rain.

STAR DREAMING PRAYER

Prayer is one of the best free gifts we receive
I asked the Ancestors for water and they gave me an ocean
I asked the Ancestors for a flower and they gave me a garden
I asked the Ancestors for a friend and they gave me all of you
If the Ancestors brings you to it, they will bring you through it

In:

Happy moments, praise the Ancestors
Difficult moments, seek the Ancestors
Quit moments, praise the Ancestors
Painful moments, trust the Ancestors
Every moment, thank the Ancestors

STAR DREAMING SONG

Mother Earth, Father Sun I love you
Grandfather and Grandmother please stay true
I promise to love you and all you have created
I thank you for the stardust and hold it in my heart
I rejoice in the gossamer lights that shine on the path
Dear family I am coming, I am coming home to the stars

STAR DREAMING MEDITATION

Before commencing your medication session, do the rituals
of Smudging/balancing /grounding/protecting and filtering
for yourself the:
- See yourself sitting quietly in a special place.
- See yourself blanketed with sparkling little starlight dragonflies.
- See them come one by one to touch the area of your heart, then kiss you on the mouth and then fly off across the earth.
- See each little starlight dragonfly flutter above each person's head - people who appear to be stumbling around in the dark.

- See a starlight dragonfly bring some light into their lives – it will help each person see clearly the false prophets and will enable them to get back on the star paths for their spiritual journey.

IN CONCLUSION

To my beautiful spirit brothers, sisters, sons, daughters and grandchildren, there is moonlight magic/medicine which should be combined with the music of love. We are the Dream-keepers who are responsible for planting the seeds (Star Seed Dreaming) of change so now is the time to step up and step out onto the star paths.

I LOVE YOU

AUNTIE BILAWARA

www.ingramcontent.com/pod-product-compliance
Lightning Source LLC
Chambersburg PA
CBHW060300030426
42335CB00014B/1775